FALL PREVENTION FOR OLDER PEOPLE:
A Survival Guide

Graham Cannard
RGN, BNS(Hons), MSc.

Published by Graham Cannard

Publishing partner: Paragon Publishing, Rothersthorpe

First published 2011

ISBN 978-1-908341-34-1

Book design, layout and production management by
Into Print

www.intoprint.net

+44 (0)1604 832149

Printed and bound in UK and USA by
Lightning Source

Dedication

This book is dedicated to Lillian Carey and Lena Kilboy; two noble and spirited ladies who taught all that knew them that advancing age is no barrier to leading an active and fulfilling life.

Acknowledgements

I owe a huge debt to my wife, Helene and my sons Lorcan and Darragh for their patience over the years that I have been away from home spreading the word on Falls Prevention. Thanks also to my two colleagues, Roy Lane and Pamela O'Brien for being the two most inspiring, expert nurses that I have encountered in my career.

To all of my nursing colleagues in the UK and Ireland and to all of the health care professionals and families around the world who have contacted me regarding falls prevention: here it is and I hope it will be of benefit.

Contents

Introduction

By choosing to read this guide you have taken the first step in helping to prevent a potentially devastating event in the life of an older person; a fall. Accidental falls account for more than seventy percent of fatal accidents in people over the age of sixty-five and with a little planning, many of these falls are preventable.

You may be reading this because you are concerned for yourself or for somebody close to you who is at risk from falling. Maybe you are reading this because somebody has already fallen and you want to reduce the risks of that from happening again. Experiencing a fall yourself or caring for somebody else who has fallen can be a very frightening and worrying experience. The future begins to look uncertain and you may not know what to do for the best. Although the consequences of falling can be very serious, it is usually the effects of repeatedly falling that pose the greatest risk and this guide is going to help you prevent this from happening.

In my thirty years as a nurse, I have worked in Accident and Emergency Departments, Orthopaedic Wards and in wards for the Care of the Older Person. I have witnessed the trauma and devastation to people who have fallen and broken bones or who have sustained head injuries. I have witnessed the worry and guilt of relatives who think they could have done more to prevent their loved one falling. In the past there probably was nothing anybody could have done because the fact is that falls used to be accepted as a natural occurrence in older people; something that had to be lived with. Thankfully in recent years a lot of work has been done to try to reduce the risks and consequences of falling. Now there is something we can do. We now know that some of the increased risk comes from the person themselves, such as age and gender. Some of these things cannot be changed but they can be recognised and acted upon. Other risks such as medications may be able to be altered. Another set of problems may be posed by the environment in which the person lives, such as poor lighting or unsafe flooring. These things are much easier to put right. Many people worry that a fall marks the beginning of a decline in health and a restricted lifestyle. In fact far from restricting independence or quality of life, this guide will help to improve independence and confidence in later years.

Whatever the circumstances, the fact that you are reading this suggests that you are concerned enough to want to do something constructive to help reduce the risk of falling. This guide is designed to enable you to understand the seriousness of older people falling, the risks that make people more prone to falling and some guidelines to help reduce those risks. If you can act before any falls occur, so much the better but it's never too late.

I suggest that you read through all sections of this guide because although some of it may seem like common-sense, there may be some things covered that you hadn't considered relevant but which may actually be very significant to your situation. At the back of this book you will find some pages for you to make a note of anything that you may need to either act upon or on which to seek further advice. If you make these notes as you go through the book then you'll be sure not to overlook anything and it will be useful if you need to talk to your G.P. or Community Nurse about it.

Chapter One

Understanding Falls

It is estimated that about one third of people over the age of sixty-five experience at least one fall each year. In the U.K. alone that is more than three million people, so it's certainly not an uncommon problem. Why then, you may ask, do we hear so little about it? There are probably a few reasons for this. First, it's only in recent years that the problem has been recognised for what it is - a major problem for some older people that can cause serious injury. Secondly, it's only since the seriousness of the problem was recognised that a lot of work has been done to try to prevent it. Accidental injury from falls costs the health services a lot of money, so it's obviously in their interest to try to prevent falls from occurring and save on the demand for hospital beds, especially in these days of cutbacks. Another reason why the problem is not talked about is the embarrassment factor. Nobody likes to fall, it can be embarrassing. If we fall, we look around and hope that nobody saw what happened and we certainly don't talk about it. But by not talking about falls doesn't mean that they will go away; while the problem stays hidden, the opportunities to put preventative measures in place are lost.

Probably the only time you'll hear of an older person falling is when they do themselves a serious injury and end up in hospital. That is because nobody likes to think of themselves as getting older, dependent and having to curtail activity. People who have had a fall often fear that if they let it be known, then their independence will be taken away from them and that they may end up in a nursing home. It's a real fear, but it's an irrational one. Let me explain why. Anybody can fall. It's not something that only happens to older people. It can happen to people of any age and for a variety of reasons. If it happens when we are younger, we look for the cause, whatever it may be and try to put it right. For example, if we trip over a child's toy left in the middle of the floor, we move the toy so it won't happen again. If we repeatedly fell over the child's toy without moving it, people close to us would start to ask questions about our ability to take care of ourselves. If we take some medication that makes us feel dizzy and we fall, we ask the doctor to change it to something that suits us better. We don't just carry on taking it, say nothing and then wonder why people close to us start to worry. We don't worry about losing independence or stop being active just because we fell. When we are younger, we don't keep quiet about it; in fact we will probably tell anybody who will listen. This is because we see the fall as a one off accident or we blame the situation. We deal with it, sort the problem out and we move on. Exactly the same principle applies if we fall when we are older. We have to deal with it and we have to move on.

The problem is that often we don't know how to deal with it. We are not quite sure how to prevent falls from happening and we think that nobody else does either. This is because people have been so busy covering up the problem that until recently very few people had bothered looking for answers. We know now that there is a lot that can be done to prevent falls as we get older, if we know where to look for help and then actually ask for that help. Admitting the problem and then acting on it is the single most important thing in reducing our risk of falling. Keeping quiet about it allows the risk to continue. Even if we decide to keep quiet about falling, it doesn't mean that nobody is going to know. There are enough tell-tale signs, especially if you know what to look for. Unexplained bruising is probably an easy sign to look out for. If a bruise is noticed, somebody is bound to ask how it happened out of genuine concern. If the explanation doesn't sound plausible, suspicions will be raised. The same happens when we are younger. For example, how many times did somebody blame a black eye on walking into a door - and how many times did you believe it? If a previously active older person suddenly starts curtailing their activities for no apparent reason, then this could suggest that they have fallen and have restricted their activities in the hope that it won't happen again. If somebody suddenly starts limping or is suddenly unable to walk it will be noticed. Obviously any of these signs could be caused by any number of things but over time a pattern begins to emerge and people will put two and two together. If it turns out that the suspicions are correct, who could blame anybody for being concerned about a friend or family member who is apparently falling and not doing anything about it? The answer is to admit the problem and to take steps to reduce it.

The effects of falls can be quite serious. Physical injury is the thing that most people think of. About one in ten people who fall each year will suffer a broken bone. Many of these people will break their hip. In older people this can be quite a serious problem as a major operation will probably be needed to fix this. Recovery can take a few months and this will further reduce activity and independence levels for a while. Some people never fully recover from a hip fracture. If somebody falls and is unable to get up again, this can cause problems even if no bones are broken. This usually happens with people who live alone. If a person is lying on the floor for more than twelve hours without being able to get up again, it is known as a 'long-lie'. This can cause respiratory problems, problems with pressure on the skin, hypothermia and several other serious effects.

Apart from the physical, is the psychological affect. Once a person has fallen, they usually become acutely aware that a problem exists and may curtail their lifestyle in an attempt to avoid further falls. If falls continue to occur, the person may impose a kind of loss of independence on themselves hoping not to fall again. We can see from this that the effects of falling can be both physical and psychological; this can alter the quality of life of an older person profoundly. It is therefore sensible to address the problem sooner rather than later.

When we are looking at ways in which we can reduce the likelihood of falling, we need to look at two main areas. The first area, which happens to be the easiest to deal with, is the physical environment. This basically means that we need to look at our living areas and make sure that they are as safe as they can be and that they pose as few obstacles as possible. It is the same idea as moving the child's toy from the middle of the floor that we mentioned before. The second area is to do with looking at our own bodies and making sure that they are functioning as well as they possibly can. We need to make sure that our physical health, where possible, does not increase our risk of falling. This area may take a little more time to deal with, but the results can be significant. Taking the time to consider these two areas and deal with any issues that may be revealed could mean the difference between living a fulfilling, active life into the future or living in fear of a fall and all of the consequences that go with it. The next chapter is going to look at the physical environment of your living area. It would be a good idea to write down in the notes pages at the end of the book, any risk factors that you notice along with any jobs that need to be done. That way you can be sure not to miss anything and to mark them off as they are completed.

Chapter Two

Hazards Around Your Home

One of the easiest and quickest ways that you can reduce your risk of falling is to make sure that your living environment is as safe as it can be. Most of the methods we will mention are easy and cheap to undertake, and mostly you will be able to do them yourself, but you may need somebody to give you a hand with some things. Do not take any unnecessary risks while carrying them out and don't be afraid to ask for help if you need it. Remember, don't hide the problem - deal with it.

Lighting

The first thing to consider is lighting. Anybody would be at a disadvantage if they had to feel their way around in the dark to get around their home. Soft mood lighting can be very relaxing and certainly has its place, as long as the main lighting in a room is bright enough to illuminate the whole area when needed. It is important to be able to see where you are going and to be able to see any obstacles in your path. The switches to all lighting should be easily accessible, not low down on the flex of a table lamp for example. A 60 watt light bulb will give off plenty of light, but be sure that the light shade can cope with it. Also, make sure that the light shade is clean. A dirty shade will significantly reduce the light from the bulb. Using an energy-saving light bulb will have the advantage of being cheaper to run in the long run and also, because they last longer, they will need changing less frequently. This may be important if you have to get somebody else to change the bulbs for you. You should make especially sure that you have adequate lighting wherever the potential dangers exist in your home. Any areas of your home that may pose special risks, stairs for example may need brighter lighting. You should also make sure that you have a bedside lamp available for night-time use so that if you have to get up, you don't have to start groping for the main light switch in the dark. Kitchens can be dangerous places, especially if you can't see properly. So make sure adequate lighting will let you see what you are doing and to see any spills on the floor. The same applies to bathrooms.

Don't forget any outside areas of your home that you may need to access in the dark. Outside steps are particularly unforgiving if you happen to trip on one as they are usually made of much harder concrete or stone. Make sure that an outside light will clearly illuminate these.

Floor Covering

Today there are many different types of floor covering to choose from and many people have a variety of different floor coverings in different rooms of their house. Each type has its own advantages. Carpets, providing that they are in good condition, offer good grip underfoot. Rubber soled slippers or shoes will not slide on a carpet and will make sure that your feet do not slide from under you. This can be important when getting up from a chair or bed. Neither do carpets become slippery when they get wet. They will offer the same grip in a wet or dry condition. Should the worst happen and you do fall, carpet will offer good protection should you hit the floor and if you are unable to get up for a while, it will be much warmer than the other kind of floor coverings. Highly patterned carpets can make it more difficult to notice any obstacle on the floor as they may blend in to the pattern, so the plainer the design, the better it is. Carpets offer significant advantages but only if they are in good condition. Frayed carpet can easily cause somebody to trip and is a positive danger. Rugs are also potential hazards for the same reason and if at all possible should not be used. If you insist on having a rug on the floor, it can be fixed to the floor with special double sided sticky tape. This will make sure the rug does not become lifted or curled up at the edges causing a trip hazard or to slide across the floor. Carpet tiles should be avoided at all costs, as over time they inevitably begin to lift causing multiple fall hazards at every lifted edge.

Lino can be useful. It usually provides good grip underfoot when it is dry, but when wet can be very dangerous and sometimes it can be very difficult to see wet areas on lino. Make sure that any joins in a piece of lino are done properly so that there is no risk of tripping over an uneven join. If necessary special tape can be used to go over any joins so that there are no uneven areas.

Ceramic tiles provide good grip when dry and there are various designs of tiles that have a non-slip surface that provide good grip even when wet. However, should a fall occur on a tiled area, your landing will be hard if you meet the floor and if you are there for any length of time, tiles are quite cold.

Timber floors or bare floorboards are very fashionable. They generally do not become slippery and providing they are well laid, should not have any edges to trip on. While not as soft as carpet, they are kinder to land on than tiles or lino should a fall occur and they are not as cold as tiles or lino. However, laminated or semi-solid flooring that looks like timber do not have the same advantages as real timber. They can be slippery when wet and are fairly cold to the touch.

These are the main types of floor covering that are likely to be found in any house. Each has its own advantages and disadvantages and as long as you are aware of these you can live safely with what you have and not have to consider replacing flooring.

Circulation Routes

These are the routes that you use to move about the house most frequently. It is important that these routes are kept free from clutter so that you will have less chance of falling over something left in your path. It is a good idea to arrange the furniture so that nothing blocks your main circulation routes or cause you to have to twist and turn like a slalom skier, as you go from room to room. Electrical flexes can be particularly hazardous if they run across the floor on a circulation route. These can provide a trip hazard as well as a fire hazard if the flex becomes damaged. You should ensure that all flexes run around the edges of the room rather than across it and that all flexes are highly visible. The use of high level plug sockets are a lot safer than the ones at skirting board level as it means that you won't have to bend or stretch to use them.

Stairs

We already mentioned that lighting on the stairwell needs to be bright enough to properly illuminate all of the stairs. A 100w equivalent energy saving bulb should provide plenty of light providing it is not surrounded by a dark coloured, or dirty shade. Stairs are a particular hazard because if you fall, you may fall a great height. The higher you fall from, the greater the injury you may suffer. So, leave nothing on the stairs. Don't leave something on the stairs 'ready to take up' next time you go. That is quite literally just placing an obstacle in your own path ready to trip yourself up. If you plan to take things upstairs next time you go, leave them on a table or chair near the foot of the stairs. They will then be out of harm's way and you won't have to bend to pick them up.

While most stairs have a banister or handrail on the outside, most don't have one against the wall. If a rail is fitted against the wall then you can hold on to both sides as you go up and down the stairs. This means that if you should fall or stumble on the stairs you have a much greater chance of being able to save yourself. If you have steps outside your house it would be worth considering getting a handrail fitted on those as well. Outside steps can be particularly hazardous in the dark, especially in icy conditions. Even with an outside light to illuminate them, it can sometimes be difficult to see the edges of the steps. If this is the case you could consider painting the edges of the steps in white paint, which will make them stand out much better, reducing the risk of falling on them.

Chairs and Seating

The problem with chairs is not in sitting on them but sitting down onto them and getting up out of them again. Most 'easy' chairs, armchairs and settees tend to be soft and accommodating and at a fairly low level. This makes them much more difficult to get up from than a dining chair, which tends to be higher and harder. The more you can 'sink in' to a chair, the more difficult you will find it to get up from. This is because the chair has more of a 'grip' on you. You will probably find that you need to shuffle your bottom forward on the seat until you get to the edge. When you get to the edge, you then have to lever yourself up on the arms of the chair, from a low level. This can be difficult if you are not as agile as you once were and is a common cause of people falling. Ideally a chair should have a seat that just touches the backs of your knees when you stand in front of it. This height of chair will need less power from your legs to stand up from. The chair should also have two arms that you can use to help lever yourself up. A carver type dining chair would actually fit these requirements nicely for most people, but of course they wouldn't be that comfortable to sit in for any length of time. What you can do, is to buy some chair raisers that fit on to each leg of an armchair and which can be adjusted to raise the chair to the right height for you. Settees can be raised in a similar fashion but unless you have very long arms you won't be able to use both arms of the settee at the same time, to lever yourself up.

It is worth mentioning a word about footstools here. While footstools can be very relaxing for the legs and feet you need to remember that they will be an obstacle in your way when you try to get into, or out of a chair. If you choose to use a stool, make sure that it is light enough for you to be able to push it out of your way with your feet from the sitting position before you actually try to stand up. You will then be able to stand and walk away from the chair without having to dodge the stool. The same principles apply to beds as for chairs. They should be at the correct height for you to exit from them easily and can be raised with chair raisers in the same way as an armchair. You could even use bricks to raise the bed a few inches.

Baths, Showers and Toilets

It is obvious that bathrooms are going to get wet because it isn't feasible to expect that anybody could keep a bathroom dry when in use. Bearing this in mind, extra care needs to be taken to make sure that even when wet the bathroom remains safe to use. Most bathroom suites are made of either plastic or enamel, both of which are smooth hard surfaces which become slippery when wet. Add to this the soap or shower gel and you have a surface as slippery as ice. To overcome this, the use of a rubber bath mat inside the bath or shower is essential. They will provide grip so that you don't slip when standing in the shower or getting into or out of the bath. A separate mat or towel placed outside the bath or shower that you can step out directly onto is also important as wet tiled floors can easily cause a slip. The use of non-slip tiles can help here also. If you find it difficult getting into or out of the bath, then you can get special bath seats that sit across the bath allowing you to sit down onto it before lifting your legs into the bath. The advantage of these seats is that you will not have to balance on one leg while you get the other leg into the bath. Grab rails on the wall and on the side of the bath are also useful for providing support and leverage to get into and out of the bath more easily. If you mainly use a shower that is in a separate cubicle, then using a shower chair in the shower, rather than standing, will help you to use the shower more safely. We will include toilets with bathrooms because in many houses today, the toilet is in the bathroom. If you find it difficult to get up and down from the toilet, you could consider getting a raised toilet seat. There are different designs available but basically they just sit on the rim of the toilet and raise the seat up by four inches or so. Grab rails on the wall are also a good idea, again to give support and leverage when sitting down onto the toilet and getting up again. If you find that you need to use the toilet frequently at night, it may be worth considering using a commode in the bedroom so that you don't need to navigate your way to the toilet in the dark. Commodes are available that look just like ordinary chairs and will not look out of place in the bedroom.

Walking Aids

Many people use walking aids, such as sticks, walking frames or tripods to help to maintain balance when walking and they can be very useful. However, it is very important that the walking aid is fitted with sound rubber ferrules (the rubber tips that come into contact with the ground). These ferrules are what prevent the walking aid from sliding from under you if you hit a wet or slippery patch on the ground. If you use an aid and have not checked the ferrule, you may be putting your trust into something that is very dangerous. Make sure you check the bottom of the ferrule and not just the sides because it is the bottom part that is going to provide the grip. The sides rarely get worn. Replacement ferrules can be obtained from many chemists very cheaply. Walking aids need to be tailored to the individual using them to make sure that the right type of aid is supplied and that they are of the correct size and height for the user. Make sure that you know how to use the aid safely. The person who supplied the aid should have given you instructions at the time but if you are unsure, check back with them.

Storage in the Home

A little planning on where to store house-hold items can make life a lot easier and safer. You should try to make sure that the items that you use most frequently are stored in the most accessible places. We tend to spend a lot of time in the kitchen for cooking, making pots of tea, putting washing into the machine and other daily tasks. Kitchens also tend to have a lot of storage areas with some being more accessible than others. It is sensible to store the items that we use frequently in the cupboards that are within easy reach. Do not make yourself over-stretch to reach items.

If you need to get an item that is not within easy reach, then use a grab stick. These have a trigger at one end of the stick and a pincer-like clamp at the other end (You often see litter collectors using them to pick up litter to save continual bending). These sticks are like an extension to your arm and mean that you will not need to climb up to get things from high cupboards, or bend down to low ones. Should you need to actually climb up to get something, never stand up on a chair. They just weren't designed for that. Instead, use a step-stool. These stools have a step underneath which can be swung down and provide a solid base to stand on. However, if you are in any way unsteady on your feet, climbing up on anything should be avoided. Step-stools can also be used to sit on, so that if you need to reach to a low cupboard, instead of bending over, you can sit down to reach the item.

Footwear

The choice of correct footwear is important because it is the part of our clothing that keeps us in contact with the ground. Shoes provide greater support for the feet than slippers. Shoes tend to be made of more rigid materials and can mean that the foot is less likely to twist when walking. Obviously any instability in footwear is going to mean instability in posture, which can lead to falls. You only need to ask somebody who wears stilettos! If possible, shoes should be of the lace-up rather than the slip-on variety. This is because slip-on shoes can get looser as they become more worn-in, and can slip off the foot nearly as easily as they slip-on. Lace-up shoes can be tightened by the laces to ensure a snug fit even when they become worn-in. If bending to tie laces is a problem, there are elastic laces available that look just like ordinary laces but will allow you to put on the shoes without having to actually untie the laces each time. These are available from many shoe shops.

Carrying Heavy or Bulky Loads

This is to be avoided if at all possible. Carrying heavy or bulky loads will alter your centre of gravity, making it much easier to topple over if you are jolted or if you bump into anything. If you need to carry something heavy, it is safer to split the load and carry a smaller load in each hand rather than a larger load in one hand. This will help to maintain your balance. When shopping for example, split the load between two bags and carry one in each hand. Carrying a large load in front of you could also diminish your field of vision meaning that you may not spot any obstacles in your path. Where possible, it is far better to split the total load and make a few trips safely rather than one hazardous trip to move the load where you need it. An example of this is bringing in fuel for an open fire. Coal is heavy and a full bucket or scuttle of coal weighs a considerable amount. Trying to carry this any distance will certainly alter your centre of gravity and your balance and increase the risk of falling. It is better to either bring in the fuel in small amounts or to get somebody else to do it for you. One suggestion is to fill a few used bread bags with coal and bring them in one or two at a time. When you need to put more coal on the fire, all you need to do is place a bag on the fire. The wrapper will burn away and the coal will then burn. Doing it this way means you are only ever handling small loads at any time.

Spectacles

Make sure you get your eyes tested regularly so that you can get glasses if you need them, or if you already wear glasses that they are of the correct prescription. If you wear glasses make sure that they are kept clean. Nobody can see where they are going properly through dirty glasses. It would be like trying to see out through a frosted glass window.

Outside the House

Getting outside the house and into the garden should be a pleasure, whether it's just to sit in the sun or to do a spot of gardening. The outside of your house should not be an obstacle course and with a little planning it needn't be. You should put as much safety planning into the garden as you would with the inside of your home, maybe even a little more. Should you happen to fall outside you need to remember that you may not easily be able to reach a telephone and you may not be able to attract attention if you need help. The paving will be hard if you do fall which could mean that you injure yourself and experience a 'long-lie' outside your house could be particularly serious in cold weather. Therefore, you need to make the garden as safe as possible so that you can continue to enjoy it.

You should check that all paved areas that you use are even. Crazy paving especially can have many uneven joints between the slabs, causing multiple trip hazards in the one area. This can be remedied with a bucket or two of cement to smooth over any areas where slabs are not flush with each other. Any steps in the garden need to be properly illuminated and the edges painted white so that they can be seen in the dark. If you are a keen gardener, then you might consider including a few raised beds. These can be built using bricks, cement blocks or old railway sleepers. If they are raised above ground level, it means that you can continue cultivation without having to bend down. You can even work the beds from a chair, or use the edges of the raised beds as a seat. Apart from reducing the likelihood of falling, it means that your back won't suffer either. If the thought of falling in the garden is a cause for concern, you should bring a mobile phone out in the garden with you just in case you need to call for help.

A Final Word

This chapter has highlighted the most common fall hazards in and around the home and has shown you that with a little planning, your home can be a safe environment in which to live. There maybe only a few minor changes that you need to make, indeed, nobody is suggesting that you have to make major changes to your familiar and comfortable surroundings. After all, your home is probably usually kept just as you like it. All that is suggested is that you remedy all the little hazards in your home so that you lessen the chance of creating one big problem for yourself. If you are safe in your home, the longer you can live an active and independent life there. When you think of it this way, the few changes you might need to make seem like an extremely good trade-off. You should use the note pages at the end of the book to write down all of the things that you've noticed that may need attention, that way you won't over-look anything.

The next chapter is going to look at how we can make sure our bodies are working as well as they can to avoid falls.

Chapter Three

Our Bodies - Risks From Within

As we mentioned before, anybody can fall. It is not confined to older people. However, it is true that the less fit and able we are, the greater is our chance of falling. As we begin to get older our bodies naturally begin to slow down a little, but age alone does not necessarily make us unfit or unhealthy. There are many older people who run marathon races every year, including people in their eighties. Equally there are many people less than a quarter of that age who would not be able to manage that. These older marathon runners have obviously kept themselves fit all their lives and the benefit of that is that they are more likely to remain physically fit into old age. The fitter you are, the less likely you are to develop long term medical problems. Luck of course plays a part too as not all medical problems can be prevented by attempting to keep physically fit, but the fitter you are, the more healthy you are likely to be.

This chapter will look at the aspects of our own bodies that may increase the risk of falling and in the next chapter we'll look at some methods of reducing the risks. There are some aspects of our bodies over which we have absolutely no control. Even though we have no control over these aspects, being aware of them and acknowledging them can be an important weapon in lessening our fall risk. First, we'll look at two factors that we cannot alter.

Gender

We have absolutely no control over our gender, we are born either a male or a female and there is nothing we can do about that. So what part does gender play in our fall risk? Many studies have shown that females have a greater fall risk than males. This could be for a variety of reasons, but is probably a combination of all of them. Firstly, women tend on average to live longer than men by about four to six years. That means four to six years of extra opportunity for women to fall than men and that during these extra years, women tend to become less fit as age increases. So the fact that women live longer puts them at a higher risk of falling than men.

In men and women of equal age, it is thought that women may experience a greater number of falls due to their higher risk of osteoporosis. Osteoporosis is a weakening of the bones that occurs naturally in both women and men as we get older, but it develops more quickly in women after the menopause because of hormonal changes. This weakening of the bones can not only mean the greater likelihood of bone injury if a fall occurs, but in certain instances, can actually be the cause of the fall itself. This is because the weakened bone cannot stand the same stresses as a strong bone and certain movements such as sudden twisting of the hip can cause the bone to break and thereby cause a fall. After the event, it can be next to impossible to tell whether the break was a result of the fall, or the cause of it.

Women tend to have a different anatomy of the pelvis to men. In women, the hips are wider to help with childbirth and this causes women to have a slightly different and less stable stance when standing to men. This lesser stability makes it easier for women to lose their balance and may therefore cause a woman to fall more easily than a man.

It has also been suggested that one of the reasons that older women may fall more than men is that the woman tends to be more physically active, doing more housework, cooking, shopping and the like, while the man tends to sit more. I'm not sure how accurate this is but maybe there is a grain of truth in it.

Age

Age plays a part in determining fall risk and there is nothing we can do to alter our age other than lie about it. In general, the older a person is, the greater their risk of falling. As we mentioned before, this is not an absolute rule. There are plenty of people of eighty who are fitter than people of twenty, but on average, the older we become, the less fit we are. The longer we live the more opportunity there is for some illness or disability to set in which will in turn, decrease our fitness levels. This decline in fitness tends to become more noticeable sometime in our sixties and will continue as our age increases unless we actively work to prevent it. A decline in general fitness means our movements tend to become less fluid and our balance can be affected making it more difficult to save ourselves if we should happen to trip. A natural slowdown in our reaction time also contributes to this.

At this point we should mention the difference between chronological age (our age counted in years) and functional age (the age at which our bodies function). There can be a huge disparity between these two ages, as in the example of the eighty year old marathon runner whose body may be functioning at the level of a forty year old. While we can't alter our chronological age, we can work on our functional age by increasing our fitness levels; and this doesn't mean that we all have to go out and start training for the London marathon! - more about that in the next chapter. The functional age is the most important in determining fall risk but that is not always easy to calculate, so to be on the safe side, we look at the chronological age.

I'm sure most people have heard the maxim "survival of the fittest". This may have some relevance in determining fall risk. It has been suggested that when people reach the age of around eighty, their fall risk may begin to decline. This is because, for a person to have reached the age of eighty, they must be fortunate enough to be relatively fit and healthy. Such people tend to have a lower fall risk than younger but less fit people. This just goes to show that age isn't everything and increasing age isn't something to get overly concerned about.

Gait

Your gait is the way that you walk and move about on your legs. As you can imagine, gait plays an important part in keeping you upright when you walk. A steady gait is when you can walk with purposeful steps, unaided and maintain a steady upright posture. This is how most people walk and it doesn't pose an increase in fall risk. As fitness begins to decline either as part of the normal aging process, or because of disability or illness, our gait can begin to change and become less stable. This is when care needs to be taken as we can often 'forget' that we are not as fit as we used to be and proceed as though we were perfectly steady when in fact we might not be.

One of the first signs to watch out for is when we become hesitant in our gait. That is to say that on standing up from a chair or a bed, we need to take a second or two to make sure we get our balance. As long as we do take the time to get our balance everything should be alright, but it does indicate that we are not as steady as we might be and care needs to be taken. Sometimes this unsteadiness on standing can be caused by a sudden drop in blood-pressure. This can be quite common and usually rectifies itself after a few seconds but if this happens on a regular basis you need to mention this to your doctor, especially if you are taking blood-pressure medication. It may mean that your doctor needs to review your medication and possibly alter the dose. If you find that you need a few seconds to steady yourself when standing, it might be sensible to make sure that you have something solid to hold onto next to the chair or bed, such as a bed-side table or another high-backed chair.

One of the most common activities to cause a fall is getting up from, or getting onto, a chair, bed or toilet, especially if you are going from one sitting position to another. An example would be getting from a bedside chair into bed. This movement from one place to another is known as a transfer. One of the reasons that this activity poses a particular risk is that not only might you have to contend with getting your balance but it also relies on muscular strength. You need good strength in your legs to lever yourself up, you need good strength in your arms to help push yourself up and you need good co-ordination to make sure that everything works together so that you land softly where you intended, either on the bed or chair: certainly not on the floor.

If you have an unsteady gait, that is have difficulty walking and maintaining your balance at the same time, then that is an obvious risk for falling. If you know that you are unsteady when walking you will need extra help to move about safely. This may be a walking stick, walking frame, or maybe just enough solid furniture or handrails for you to be able to hold onto whilst moving around. There are aids available to keep you mobile and safe at the same time. If you think that you may need help, contact your G.P. or Practice Nurse who will be able to refer you to the right person. Never be too proud to use a walking aid if you need it. It's far better to live an active and independent life with a walking aid than to be bed-bound with a broken hip and totally dependent on others, trust me on this one. Now we'll look at some of the risk factors that we can do something about.

Medication

As we get older, the chance increases of developing a medical condition that requires medication. Sometimes we only need to take medication for a fixed length of time, on the other hand we may need to take certain medications for the rest of our lives. Either way, there are certain medications that can increase our risk of falling even though they may be necessary to keep us otherwise healthy. One of the greatest risks comes from having to take a combination of medications. The more medications we take, the greater the risk of medications interacting with each other. Certain medications do not mix well with each other and can cause unwanted side-effects. In other cases some medications interact with each other to make the effect of one of the medications greater than it would have been on its own. Depending on which medications are taken, this could possibly increase drowsiness or unsteadiness or in some other way make us less able to move about safely. Prescription medications that can cause drowsiness usually have a label attached to the bottle or box indicating this fact. Your Doctor will have course considered this and kept you on a minimum of medication but if you feel that your medication may be in some way causing you to be less steady when walking or moving about, it is important that you discuss this with him or her. I should stress here that on no account should you alter your medication or stop taking it without first discussing it with your doctor or nurse. You may do yourself far more harm by not taking medication that is vital to your health. There are many different medications that may increase your risk of falling to some degree. The most common ones are medications that might alter your level of alertness and medications that control high blood pressure, although these are not the only ones. Diuretics (water tablets) for example can increase fall risk if you frequently have to use the toilet, especially at night.

If you are taking medication that may reduce your level of alertness, then it is possible that your gait will be affected in a similar way to if you have taken alcohol. You may fail to take adequate care when moving about and this will cause an obvious increase in your risk of falling. This would be true for anybody regardless of age, but if you already have an increased fall risk, these medications could make it worse. These medications will cause your reaction time to be lessened, meaning it will take you longer to react if you should trip or begin to fall. Sleeping tablets or sedatives are two such types of medication, so if you need to take these, you need to make sure that all other risks are at an absolute minimum. You also need to remember that alcohol will greatly enhance the affect of these medications and should be avoided whilst taking sleeping tablets or sedatives. Alcohol can also react badly with other medications so it would be wise to check with your doctor or pharmacist if it's OK to take a drink.

Medication to reduce high blood pressure may also cause problems in some people. The problem arises if the medication is too 'strong' and causes the blood pressure to drop too far. Sometimes the medication may cause you to feel lightheaded, especially when standing up from a sitting or lying position. If this happens, then talk to your doctor. It may mean that a change of medication will sort this problem out. However, if you find that this is happening to you, you will probably find that if you get up slowly, bit by bit, the problem will be far less. For example, when getting out of bed, first sit up in bed and wait a few seconds. Then sit on the edge of the bed and wait another few seconds, then slowly stand up. This gives the body time to adjust.

Although we've looked at two common types of medication, these are not the only types that could increase your fall risk. If you are on any type of medication, it is advisable that you get your doctor to review them periodically so that you don't end up taking medication that you may not actually need anymore. The more medication you are on, the greater the risk for the drugs to have unwanted side-effects. You must also consider any medications that you have bought 'over the counter'. These medications can also interact with prescribed medications so it is very important that you tell your doctor if you are taking any 'over the counter' medication.

One last point on medication: It has been found that grapefruit juice can enhance the affect of some types of medication. This may mean that the medication is having more of an effect than is required and can therefore cause problems. Your pharmacist can advise you on whether it is safe to take grapefruit juice with your medications.

Sight and Hearing

A deficit in the sense of sight or hearing can be a cause of an increased risk of falling. It is fairly easy to see why impaired eyesight can cause a fall. If we can't see where we are going or what obstacles are in our way, we are asking for trouble. It is so easy to trip on something that we cannot see. It is possible that poor vision in fact causes more falls due to loss of balance than simply tripping over an obstacle. This is because sight also plays a big part in maintaining balance. The messages from our eyes are constantly sent to our brain so that we can tell where exactly we are in relation to our surroundings. These messages along with messages sent from our inner ear are vital for us to maintain balance. For example, skiers buried in avalanches are effectively blind. All they can see is white all around them. They cannot tell which way is up or which way is down because it all looks the same. If they can't tell which way is up, they cannot help to dig their way to the surface and risk death because of it. Skiers caught in this situation are advised to dribble saliva from their mouths, which will fall down due to gravity and from this they can work out which way is up and start digging. In the same way, if we are not receiving adequate information from our eyes, our bodies have a much more difficult job knowing which way is up. This can mean that we may not be able to maintain balance and we fall. For this reason it is important that regular eye tests are carried out by your optician to make sure that you get glasses if you need them, or if you already wear glasses that the prescription is still adequate. Sight naturally changes with age, so the glasses that were suitable two years ago, may not be suitable now. Regular eye tests are the only way to make sure that the prescription is still right for your eyesight. As mentioned before, if you do wear glasses, it is vitally important that you keep them clean. Trying to see where you are going through a pair of dirty glasses is like trying to drive a car through a frosted up windscreen. You just wouldn't do it. It's an obvious point, but one which many people ignore.

Hearing is another sense which can play a part in increasing the fall risk in some people, although it is probably more of interest to those who are carers for somebody else. If you are caring for somebody who has a risk of falling, you may need to talk to them about certain risks, such as to watch out for a vacuum cleaner whilst the housework is being done, or to watch out for an icy path in the garden. If somebody is very frail, you may just need to tell them to ask for help if they need to get up from a chair or to go to the toilet. We need to be sure that what we have said is actually heard by the other person. If they don't hear the warning, they obviously will not act on it. As we get older hearing does tend to become less acute, but when hearing loss becomes a problem, carers need to make sure that what they say is actually heard, as it could mean the difference between a safe environment and a hazardous one. So if you need to give a warning to somebody you are caring for, it is a good idea to check with them that they actually heard you. If hearing loss is a severe problem, talk to your doctor. There may be simple treatments that may improve the situation or aids that may help.

History of Falling

It is widely recognised that once somebody has fallen, this is a strong indicator that they may fall again. This is because if somebody has fallen once, it shows that there is a strong likelihood that some of the risk factors we have been talking about are present. If we don't take some action to reduce those risk factors, they will remain present to cause another fall. This is why it is so important that if you have fallen, you need to look for appropriate help to prevent it from happening again. Ignoring the problem will not make it go away. You can fall once and learn from it, or you can ignore it and just wait for it to happen again. It really is as simple as that.

The location where the fall actually happened can also be an important factor to note. If somebody falls in their own home, then immediate action needs to be taken. This is because we are all familiar with our own homes, we know the layout like the back of our hand and we know all the potential hazards. We should be able to negotiate our way around our home with relative safety by avoiding those hazards we know about. If we can't do this in what should be the safest area then we need to take action to remedy the situation. If we fall outside of our own home, in the garden for example, then although the layout and hazards are probably familiar to us, there is less we can do to control the situation. We can't stop ice from forming in the winter, we can't stop grass from growing and hiding hazards in the lawn and we can't stop the wind from blowing obstacles around. So while falling in our own familiar garden can be a serious event, we are sometimes limited in the controls that we can put in place. The hazards we can't control, we need to be aware of so that they can be avoided. The difference between falling inside our home and falling in the garden is that we can control the environment inside, but not outside. We can expect the inside of our home to be the same tomorrow as it is today; we cannot say this about the garden. Therefore when using the garden we need to be cautious of every potential hazard. The other scenario is when we fall outside of our home environment altogether. We can neither control, nor be aware of, all of the hazards that we may encounter in the street or somebody else's home and neither can we be expected to be. If we have an increased risk for falling then we need to take extra care when outside of our own environment and expect the unexpected.

Medical History

Falling is not a medical problem in itself. Falls however may be caused by an existing medical problem. As we get older, the chances become greater that we will at some time, acquire a medical problem. This is an unfortunate fact of life, but some medical conditions can heighten your risk of falling because of the way our body reacts. We already mentioned deteriorating eyesight as one risk factor but there are many others. It all boils down to the symptoms caused by the particular medical condition and how those symptoms may limit our ability to remain upright. Any medical conditions that may reduce muscle strength, alter gait or alter the level of consciousness may play a part in increasing our risk of falling. There are a lot of conditions that can cause one or more of these symptoms, so it's beyond the scope of this guide to go into every one of them but most people will know if their medical condition could cause any of these symptoms and if they don't, then it would be a good idea to talk to the GP or nurse to find out. It is important to remember that some medical conditions can go unrecognised and undiagnosed, especially if their onset is very gradual. An example of this would be diabetes. Many people who have diabetes don't know it. It is often picked up on a visit to the doctor during routine screening or as part of tests for something else. Diabetes usually has a slow but gradual onset and people often don't realise there is anything wrong apart from a set of vague symptoms which they may put down to simply being tired. So on a visit to the doctor about 'feeling tired all the time', tests may reveal diabetes as part, or all, of the problem. Diabetes is a serious disease if not properly controlled and if not properly treated, can cause confusion, coma and in rare cases death. The reason I've used this as an example is that just because we don't know that we have a medical problem doesn't necessarily mean that one doesn't exist and that problem may be the cause of falls. If somebody is falling regularly for no obvious reason, it is essential that they are checked out by a doctor because a hidden medical problem may be the cause. Treatment of that medical problem may be all that is required to dramatically reduce that person's fall risk and this another very good reason why people who are experiencing falls should not hide the problem. If they do, then they may be hiding a lot more than they may realise, at great cost to their health and lifestyle. It goes without saying that for any medical condition, it is wise to follow your doctor's advice regarding treatment and to ask .about anything you may be unsure about.

Mobility

Mobility refers to how well a person can move about. Full mobility is when a person can move about to do all they need to do, without the need of any aids. For example, somebody with full mobility would be able to walk around the shops to do their own shopping, move freely and easily around their home and manage stairs easily. Somebody with full mobility would have a low fall risk by virtue of the fact that they are obviously fit enough to be able to get around, but there is a word of caution. If somebody is fit enough to move around easily, then they have plenty of opportunity to encounter hazards that may cause a fall, especially if they are in an unfamiliar environment. So because a person has no difficulty getting about doesn't necessarily mean that they are immune to falls. They just need to keep alert to any hazards that they may encounter.

Some people need to use a walking aid of some sort such as a walking stick, walking frame or tripod. The use of these aids can improve a person's mobility, but the fact that they need to use a walking aid in the first place indicates that they are experiencing some difficulty in walking safely and that in itself indicates an increased risk of falling. Another difficulty associated with walking aids is that unless they are correctly measured to suit the user and maintained properly, they can actually be a hazard in themselves. A poorly maintained walking aid can actually cause falls rather than prevent them. A walking aid needs to be at the correct height for the user and should have been measured by the person that supplied the aid. If you are unsure about this, you should contact your practice nurse, community nurse or physiotherapist, who will be able to help you. As mentioned before, it is also vital that the rubber tip (ferrule) at the bottom of the walking aid is in good condition in order to prevent the aid from sliding on slippery surfaces. The area of the ferrule to check is the underside, the part that comes into contact with the ground. If it is worn at all, then it needs to be replaced. Many larger chemists stock replacement ferrules.

Restricted mobility is when a person's ability to move about is compromised. They may not be able to move very far, perhaps being housebound. They may not be able to manage stairs or may only be able to move with support of furniture or another person. People who have restricted mobility are at the highest risk for falls because they are not steady on their feet and may not be able to save themselves if they do begin to fall. People who have restricted mobility can find day to day tasks very challenging and need to make sure that all other risks are reduced to an absolute minimum. With some careful planning of the environment and the way they carry out activities, people with restricted mobility can lead reasonably active lives and remain reasonably safe.

You would imagine that people who are bed or chair bound would have no risk of falling, but this is not quite true. It is quite common for people to fall out of bed or a chair, especially if they are a little confused and think that they have full mobility when they don't. If somebody who usually stays in the bed or chair forgets that they can no longer walk unaided, and attempts to get up, it is almost inevitable that they will fall. The only place that somebody can not fall from is the floor! So if somebody that you care for is bed or chair bound, do not assume that they will not be able to fall.

Summary

We have looked at the eight most common risk factors that may increase falls; gender, age, gait, sight and hearing, fall history, medications, medical history and mobility. Any of these can increase a person's fall risk and need to be assessed. If you notice any of the factors may be affecting you or somebody that you care for, it would be a good idea to note them down now in the notes pages at the end of the guide. This will help to remind you that you may need to discuss some of the risks with your doctor, and you can bring this list with you so that nothing is over-looked.

In the next chapter, we are going to look at some of the ways we can prevent falls from happening and what to do if they do happen.

Chapter Four

Important Fall Reduction Measures

Before you read any further, it is important to stress that as long as somebody is moving around there is always the slight chance that they may fall. There can never be a guarantee that falls can be prevented 100% of the time unless somebody chooses to lie flat on the floor and not move; this is the only place from which there is nowhere left to fall. Obviously nobody is going to do that, so the plan is to make sure the risk of falling is reduced as far as possible, while still maintaining an acceptable quality of life. The quality of life issue is very important to consider. While nobody wants to fall, nobody wants their lifestyle curtailed to such an extent that life loses its sparkle. It's important to be able to strike a balance between maintaining safety and still being able to enjoy life. Certain risks may need to be taken to maintain a meaningful quality of life. If those risks are acceptable to the individual concerned and they fully understand the risk they are taking, then they need to be supported in those decisions. Nobody has the right to make those decisions on somebody else's behalf and then impose them, it doesn't work anyway. Even when somebody may be suffering from a period of confusion, trying to impose restrictions is fraught with difficulties. They may not understand what is being said, or they may not remember. This can give the care giver a false sense of security because they may think the individual concerned will comply with the restrictions, when in reality they may not. If somebody is at an increased risk of falling and they are not willing or able to comply with restrictions to their activity, the best way is to work with them if possible to come to a compromise. For example, if somebody insists on going up and down the stairs when there is a clear danger to their safety, a compromise may be to get them to agree to ask for help when they need to use the stairs, or to install a stair-lift. That way they can still use the stairs but the risks have been minimized. With a bit of inventiveness, many risks can be minimized and may be the best we can do if we are trying to protect somebody who is unwilling or unable to accept help. Remember, you can get help and advice from your practice nurse, district nurse or occupational therapist if you run into difficulties.

It is important at this point to mention the use of restraint. The facts are quite simple. The use of restraint is an ineffective, dangerous and ethically very questionable measure to take. In the past such items as cot-sides, harnesses, baffle locks and 'geriatric chairs' have been used to try to prevent people from falling. The rationale was that if we could prevent somebody from moving then they couldn't fall. The trouble with this is that these out-dated interventions actually caused far more harm than they prevented. Cot-sides for example cannot prevent a person from trying to get out of bed. What they can do is increase agitation in somebody who is fighting against a barrier to get up and they also will effectively increase the height that a person is going to fall if they do manage to negotiate their way over the top of the cot-side. Harnesses, straps or belts that tie a person into a bed or chair will not only increase agitation but they can also cause physical injury if the person is fighting to get out of them. More than one person has been killed by these devices when they managed to slip down the chair in an effort to get free and were strangled by the strap or belt. Physical restraint greatly increases a person's risk of harm and should not be undertaken in any circumstances. The use of chemical restraint by the use of medication will equally not prevent falls. It is highly likely that it will increase a person's fall risk and should therefore never be used for the purpose of fall prevention. As we mentioned before, increasing somebody's level of sedation, will only make them more unsteady and cannot hope to prevent falls. It is partly for these reasons and partly for legal reasons that hospitals and nursing homes do not use such restraints and cannot accommodate any requests to do so from relatives who may mistakenly think they will help.

Nutrition

Maintaining a good, balanced diet is important when thinking about fall prevention for two reasons. The first is that a diet rich in calcium and vitamin D will help to maintain strong healthy bones, especially for people who have a degree of osteoporosis. Osteoporosis is the gradual loss of bone tissue associated with aging, especially in women. A diet rich in calcium, which we get mainly from dairy products and fish with edible bones (like sardines) helps to maintain bone strength. Our bodies also need vitamin D to help absorb the calcium from the diet. Some foods such as fortified milk have added vitamin D, but our body can manufacture its own vitamin D by exposing our skin to sunlight. Exposing our face and arms to daylight occasionally for about fifteen minutes will be enough to supply our requirement of vitamin D. This is especially important in people who may be housebound, who may not normally get this daily exposure. Sitting by an open window or door when the weather permits would overcome this problem and using fortified milk or other foods will help to correct any deficit.

Strong bones will not only help protect against any fractures if a fall should happen, but it may also help to prevent falls in people with osteoporosis. This is because the bones of people with osteoporosis become more brittle and may not be able to withstand the strain of a sudden twisting movement to the hip for example. This can mean that a sudden twist of the hip may be all that is required to cause the hip to fracture and thereby cause a fall. After the event it is often difficult to tell if the fracture was as a result of the fall or the cause of it, so it is wise to try to make sure than our bones stay in the healthiest condition they can be in.

Apart from calcium and vitamin D, our bodies also need enough proper nutrition to keep everything else in our body working as it should. We need carbohydrates for energy, protein for repair and growth, some fats to help absorb vitamins and of course adequate fluids to keep everything going. A lack of fluids can lead to dehydration, which if not corrected can cause confusion, disorientation and unsteadiness. This will obviously increase somebody's fall risk. A balanced diet will help to maintain our bodies in good overall health and maintain a healthy weight. We all hear everyday about the growing problem of obesity and the harmful effects this can have on our health in general. Being overweight will reduce fitness levels and can make moving around much more difficult. On the other hand, being underweight can equally have its problems. If you are not eating enough to provide the energy you need, your muscles will become weakened and this may lead to a fall. In addition to this, should a fall occur you will have far less 'padding' around you to help prevent fractures. Maintenance of a healthy weight will ensure you are in the best position to avoid falls and also to cope with them should they occur.

A word here about alcohol would be a good idea. Alcohol is a depressant. It slows reaction times and can remove inhibitions and this is precisely why there is a drink driving limit. If alcohol can inhibit the ability to drive, it can also inhibit the ability to move around safely on foot, hence the expression 'footless' for somebody who is inebriated. If alcohol can make a normally steady person fall, think how much more easily it can cause a fall in somebody who already has an increased risk. If somebody with an increased fall risk takes alcohol, then it should be done in sensible amounts and in an environment that is as safe as it can be. Ideally, the person should not be drinking when alone. It would be far better to take a drink in company so that if assistance is required it is readily available.

Alcohol can also interact with many medications, making their effect much more pronounced, which can be a problem especially with medication that alters the level of alertness such as sleeping tablets. Be very aware of this and check with your doctor or pharmacist if you are unsure about the safety of combining medication with alcohol.

Exercise

Exercise can help to increase our general level of overall fitness, improve muscle strength, improve balance and co-ordination and may help to prevent osteoporosis. That's a great prevention package in itself and the even better news is that it shouldn't be an ordeal. One word of caution: if you are not used to taking much exercise, or if you have a medical condition, then it is wise to consult your doctor before beginning an exercise programme.

Exercise should not hurt or make you feel bad, so take it easy and gradually build up your fitness. If you start to feel uncomfortable while exercising, stop and consult your doctor. Remember, the aim of this kind of exercise is to build suppleness and general fitness, not to train for the next Olympics. Everything should be gentle and easy. Walking, swimming, gardening and housework are all physical exercise. In fact activity that keeps you moving will help you to keep fit, but there are other exercises that can help to improve this even further. Check to see if any local groups offer exercise programmes that you could join. Some local health care providers provide exercise classes either on their own or as part of a more extensive fall prevention programme, so it would be worth enquiring if there are any classes in your area. The important point to remember is to start slowly and gently and gradually increase your effort as your general fitness improves.

If you are unable to join in an organised fitness programme or are unable to manage housework or gardening, there are still exercises that you can do at home. If you are able to stand safely and steadily, then repeating some of the following exercises five to ten times a day will help to improve fitness and suppleness. Just make sure before you start that you have a clear space around you except, maybe, for a high-backed chair or other solid surface that you can hold on to for balance if necessary.

- Stand, feet apart, swing arms around in circles.
- Do imaginary 'bell-ringing' exercises.
- Drop alternate shoulders from side to side.
- Bend to touch alternate toes (or as near as you can safely get).
- Stand up on tip-toe and rock slowly back onto heels.
- Stand on tip-toe, bend legs and slowly straighten up.

If you are not confident about being able to do the standing exercises, then there are some alternatives that you can do from a chair, again make sure you have space around you.

- Turn head from left to right and up and down.Hunch shoulders and relax

- Stretch arms over your head and lower slowly to sides.

- Reach down over the sides of the chair, alternate sides.

- Clasp hands together and lift over head.

- Lift legs up and down alternate sides.

- Stamp feet on floor.

- Rock feet from heel to toe on floor.

After you have completed the exercises just take a minute to relax before you continue on with your usual schedule. These types of exercise, apart from improving suppleness, can also improve balance and that will certainly help with preventing falls and weight-bearing exercises such as walking will also help to guard against osteoporosis.

Exercise can be a part of most people's daily activity one way or another and it will help not only to maintain overall fitness, but it will also help to reduce the risk of falling. The other benefit is that should a fall occur, increased fitness may mean that it is possible to save yourself before you actually meet the floor. Even if the fall results in you meeting the floor, being fit will enable you to get up more easily and if an injury should occur, that you should be able to recover more quickly. That should be enough to convince most people to keep moving in order to help themselves maintain their safety and independence.

Surveillance

We are not talking about undercover police operations here. Surveillance just means 'close observation'. Surveillance will not necessarily prevent people from falling but it will ensure that help is available should a fall occur. Observation of somebody who has an increased risk of falling is important for several reasons. If somebody does fall, it is important that somebody is available to provide whatever assistance may be required. Equally as important is the fact that an older person who may have an increased fall risk will undoubtedly feel more confident and reassured to know that that help is available. However, unless somebody is aware that assistance is required it may not be provided. This can be a matter of life or death in some circumstances. Of course, everybody will have different needs and requirements and the level of observation that suits one person may be seen as obtrusive or interfering to another. It is important to try to get the level of observation right, both in terms of the amount of observation and the way it is delivered.

Everybody has a right to privacy; nobody would like to think they are under constant observation with somebody else watching their every move. Therefore, it is important that the level of observation offered is acceptable to all parties, most importantly, to the person with the increased falls risk. There are many ways of providing this observation or help and in this case surveillance doesn't necessarily mean having to physically keep watch over somebody, it just means devising a method of knowing when help is required and then providing that help.

Where somebody with an increased fall risk lives with somebody else who is reasonably fit and healthy, this provides the closest and surest surveillance. If the person falls there will be somebody on site to provide assistance or to call for further help if required. However, in reality, many older people live alone and many prefer it this way, so there isn't constant surveillance present. In these situations alternative methods of surveillance need to be put in place.

One method of doing this is to arrange for somebody to call in a couple of times a day to make sure everything is OK, a neighbour perhaps, or a friend or relative who is reasonably close by. Ideally whoever is going to call in should have a key so that if they need to get in to the house, they can. Another way of maintaining surveillance is to arrange with a neighbour to watch out for curtains being pulled at a certain time each morning and evening. Should they notice that the curtains haven't been drawn by a certain time they could come and check that everything is OK. If there is no neighbour available to do this then a friendly milkman or postman may agree to help.

Beyond this physical surveillance there are alarm devices available. These can be helpful if there is nobody available to call in, or even as an addition to this. There are various organisations that provide alarm pendants that are worn around the neck of the vulnerable person. Should a fall (or any other emergency) occur, pressing a button on the alarm will alert a call centre, who will in turn alert a prearranged contact person. If the call centre fails to make contact with this person they will alert the emergency services. Some of these alarm systems are run by local authorities, some by charitable organisations and some by private companies. You should be able to find out who provides this service in your area from your local health centre or local authority.

There are other types of alarm devices that are designed to alert somebody else in the house that a vulnerable person may be putting themselves at risk. These types of alarm can be useful if somebody who needs help when moving around is not able to call for help before moving. One such alarm, known as an Ambularm ™, is a device about the size of a matchbox which is worn just above the knee attached to a soft legband. When the wearer moves the leg from the horizontal to the vertical position, as they would when getting out of a bed or chair, the alarm is triggered to let others within earshot know that the wearer is moving into the upright position. This can be especially useful at night or when the vulnerable person is in another room to the carer as it allows the carer to get to the person quickly before any harm is done. Ambularms ™ have been successfully used in hospitals and nursing homes to alert staff quickly that somebody may be at risk. There are also other types of alarm available that can warn a carer that somebody with a high fall risk is moving into a dangerous position. These types of alarm are obviously only suitable for people who have somebody else living with them or in constant attendance.

When considering any type of alarm device it is important that the cooperation and agreement of the wearer is obtained. This is important because it would be a serious invasion of privacy if such a device were imposed upon somebody against their will. There will be instances where it may not be possible to obtain agreement because the wearer is not able to understand or to give their informed consent. In these instances it needs to be considered whether the greater benefit will served to the person by wearing the alarm or not. This is a personal decision and the rights and wrongs will vary from person to person. The aim is to provide the best possible quality of life to the vulnerable person and whichever action will provide this is the right way to go.

Having surveillance in place will ensure that help is available if a fall should occur but will rarely be able to prevent a fall. This is an important point to remember. If somebody else lives with a vulnerable person and they happen to fall, no blame or guilt should attach to that person. There is no way that surveillance on its own can prevent a fall unless the vulnerable person is being watched for every minute and every second of the day and night and that isn't feasible. The same applies to older people who may live in a nursing home or be in hospital. The staff in hospitals and nursing homes equally cannot prevent a fall by surveillance alone because the only place in either setting where observation is constant is in an Intensive Care Unit. In every other part of a hospital, or in nursing homes, staff are required to care for many people at the same time. They cannot be in every room or ward at the same time. They cannot keep constant watch over somebody. How many people would feel comfortable knowing that their every move was being watched anyway? It is reasonable to expect hospitals and nursing homes to have fall prevention measures in place and that the environment is safe, but just as at home, these measures are not a guarantee that falls will not occur. Usually, the safest place for a person at risk of falls is their own home, providing the environment is safe. They are familiar with it and all the hazards within. This is not so in a strange environment, where falls will be more common. It is therefore a mistake to think that somebody would be better off in a nursing home simply because they may be at risk of falls. Of course, there are plenty of reasons why a nursing home may be an appropriate place to live, but falls alone is not one of them unless absolutely no kind of surveillance in the home is possible.

What to do if a Fall Should Occur

First, don't panic, just lie still and gather your thoughts for a few moments. If there is somebody else in the house or within ear-shot, call out for help. If there is nobody around, the first thing you need to do is to check for any injury. Slowly and gently start to move your arms and legs. Notice any pain on movement or if moving your arms and legs causes pain anywhere else such as your back or neck. If you have severe pain, use any alarm device to call for help and remain still until help arrives. If you don't have an alarm device, see if you can gently pull yourself towards a telephone and call for help by dialling 999 or 112 and asking for the ambulance service. Give your name and address and explain what has happened. Follow any instructions the emergency service gives you and wait for help.

If you feel that you have no severe pain or injury, slowly roll onto your stomach, all the time checking for pain. Gradually get onto your hands and knees and crawl slowly to a chair. Put your hands onto the seat of the chair and raising one leg at a time, gradually lift yourself to a sitting position on the chair. Do all of this slowly and gradually. This is important because if you do have an injury you don't want to make it any worse, or worse still, to fall again. When you are on the chair, check again for any injuries. If you do have any injury, especially if you have hit your head, immediately call for help from family, neighbours or the emergency services. It is important that any injury, as well as the cause of the fall is checked out. Remember, don't ignore it, and don't keep quiet about it. Next time you may not be so lucky.

If you are unable to get up, try to manoeuvre yourself onto a soft, warm surface like a carpet. If there is something that you can reach to cover yourself, use it because you can become cold very quickly lying on the floor. If you think you may have to wait a while for help it is important that not only do you keep warm, but to relieve pressure on the bony parts of your body every half an hour. Try shifting your weight a fraction from your hips, buttocks and shoulders. This will help to prevent pressure sores from developing. If you have been able to set up some sort of surveillance and you know that somebody will be checking on you or watching out for your curtains being drawn, then you know that help will arrive at that time. This is why surveillance is so important.

Chapter 5

Further Help

Hopefully this guide will have answered some of your questions about falls and fall prevention, however, everybody is different and you may have questions or a personal set of circumstances that haven't been covered here. If so, there are plenty of other places that can give you further information and help. The first port of call should be your GP. Your GP will know you and be able to provide all the medical information that you need. They will also be able to refer you to a Practice Nurse, Community Nurse, Physiotherapist or other health professional as required. Your GP practice may have information on further services available locally.

Other organisations exist that can also offer help and advice, although they won't know you personally, they can offer general advice. There are also national organisations that can provide information. The following organisations can be contacted by telephone; they also have websites on the internet.

NHS Direct   0845 4647
www.nhsdirect.nhs.uk

Age Concern   020 8765 7200
vvww.ageconcem.org.uk

Help the Aged 02072781114
www.helptheaged.org.uk

ROSPA   01212482000
www.rospa.com

Your local authority and local health authority may also have information available and may be able to give information on local fall prevention services.

Apart from all of the above, the most important people to get help from are family, friends and neighbours if you have any nearby. These people will know you and your circumstances and may be able to provide help with any jobs that may need to be done. They may also be able to provide support and surveillance. However, they will be able to do none of this if you don't mention your concerns. It is vitally important that if you have fallen or if you think you may be at risk, that you seek help from somebody. Failure to address this will inevitably lead to the problem becoming worse and putting yourself at risk of serious injury, restricted lifestyle or other serious consequences. Don't wait for the issue to become a problem, deal with it now. Remember, you are in the company of more than 10 million other people aged over 65 years who are all in the same boat; and that's a lot of people.

Now you have read this guide, you need to act on anything that you've written down in the notes pages. Do it now. Don't leave it until tomorrow or next week. If you need to make an appointment to see your doctor, do it now. If you need to paint white lines on your outside steps, go and get the paint. Do whatever you need to do to stay safe.

About one third of people over the age of sixty-five will fall each year. Make sure you're not one of them!

NOTES

NOTES

ACTION PLAN

Lightning Source UK Ltd.
Milton Keynes UK
UKOW06f0817070617
302831UK00021B/403/P